Pra

"*The Tru*... ...*sex helped me* see sex in a new way. I thought it would be stuff I already knew and a waste of time, but it turned out to be the exact opposite of what I thought. Hearing about the predator vs the protector really surprised me. The book made me realize sex has a whole lot more risks than I thought. I would definitely recommend this book to my friends."

—AKEEM, AGE 13

"*The Truth About Sex* is a **gamechanger!** Jackie Brewton has written a challenging and inspiring book, with stories from teen guys that are educational and intriguing. I found myself wishing someone would have shared this book with me when I was a hormone driven 16-year-old boy, thinking I was a man! It will inspire any young man who reads it to live with character, integrity and chase his purpose instead of pleasure!"

—YANNIK MCKIE, FATHER, PASTOR AND AUTHOR OF *LIVING IN PURPOSE*

"**Thank you for writing** *The Truth About Sex*. I loved the honesty of the conversations and learning that boys are valuable too. I was glad to read that other teen guys were feeling some of the same things that I do. It lets me know that the way I feel about waiting is okay."

—MATTHEW, 15

"*The Truth About Sex* is **excellent!** If young men actually take the time to read and internalize the information in this book, there is no way they will have the same thought process afterward. I love how it incorporates student dialogue, student letters, and thought-provoking questions at the end of each chapter. It not only teaches young men about sex, but more importantly about their purpose and identity as a man."

—CHRIS CANNON, FATHER AND AUTHOR OF *THE MYSTERY OF MANHOOD*

"The Truth About Sex is amazing and very well-written with important information that's impactful for young men in my generation. I'm glad it includes input from guys my age whose stories made me think about how the decisions I make today can impact my life and others' years down the line. If I'm ever in a situation where I have to make a decision regarding sex, the teachings from this book will be at the forefront of my mind."

—BRADLEY, 16

"The Truth About Sex was a wonderful read. The letters from students are stunning, yet honest glimpses into the thoughts, feelings, and pressures of teenage boys. Every parent should want to stand at this 'window' and look in. What I 'saw' frightened me some, but inspired me more to reach my son in this life-changing area. I am now motivated to ask that we read this guide together. As a pastor, a parent, a Behavior Interventionist, and one who believes in U-turns, I whole-heartedly recommend this book. It says to teen boys, 'You are valuable; therefore, you can make choices that recognize your value, even if you're made different choices in the past.'"

—MICHELLE SIMPKINS, MOM OF TEEN GUY, PASTOR

"The Truth About Sex is full of valuable information and teaches teen guys the best way to live without sex. It also reveals many of the misguided reasons teen guys have sex. I like that it gives stories of actual teen guys and the chapters are not too long to read."

—XAVIER, 19

"The Truth About Sex will help me with future dialogue with my teenage son and I would recommend it to every parent of a pre-teen or teen son. There is something in it for all and no stone was left unturned. Young men will benefit just knowing the questions they secretly have are also on the minds of just about every other young man; but they are either too embarrassed to ask or too proud to admit that they just don't know certain things. I also love that it is written to young men and not at them."

—TRAVIS STOVES, FATHER OF TEEN GUY

"*The Truth About Sex* is a great book that really speaks to pre-teen and teen boys. It gives great reasons as to why we shouldn't have sex at our age. I liked the self-reflection questions included. They help you ask yourself important questions you might not have thought of if you didn't read the book, which can really help someone who needs it now and help me in the future. I would read this book again and recommend it to my peers."

—AUBREY, 12

"As a father of two sons and two daughters and also a health educator, I found *The Truth About Sex* to be a perfect tool for guiding conversations about sexual activity and a source of clarity that not all teen boys are sexually active and some actually decide to wait. The real stories and the reflection questions provide a great launch pad for having 'the talk' within a large group setting, small group, or one-on-one conversations. This book should be in the personal library of every student, parent, and educator."

—BRODERICK SANTIAGO, FATHER,
PASTOR & HEALTH EDUCATOR

"I like how *The Truth About Sex* has testimonials from the peers of the readers where they can hear their own struggles from those they relate to best. I think that's a very effective strategy. The questions at the end of each chapter are thought-provoking and challenges teen guys to consider their thoughts and actions."

—DEREK Q. SANDERS, AUTHOR
OF *MAKING SENSE OF LOVE*

"*The Truth About Sex* is absolutely amazing! The author brings in her experience with speaking to teens and is able to help boys understand the consequences of their actions in a way that makes sense. One thing that the youth complain about is that sometimes their parents or adults will tell them not to do something, but can't give them reasons why. *The Truth About Sex* provides the why. Each chapter gives great discussion topics that go beyond sex. The book is framed in a way to help teens think future minded and about setting goals for themselves. As a single mom, the conversations that I was able to have with the aid of this book were priceless. My son and I read it together; we both enjoyed it. He didn't see it as punishment or unnecessary, but very helpful."

—Charlene Clark, Mom & Teacher

THE TRUTH ABOUT SEX

REAL STORIES FROM TEEN GUYS LIKE YOU

JACKIE BREWTON

Copyright © 2022 by Jackie Brewton
All Rights Reserved
Published by HLB Press
www.hlbpress.com

All rights reserved. No part of this book may be reproduced in any form or by any means, electronic or mechanical, including photocopying or recording, or by any information and storage retrieval system, without written permission of the publisher.

ISBN: 978-0-9973405-3-2 (paperback)
ISBN: 978-0-9973405-4-9 (eBook)
ISBN: 978-0-9973405-5-6 (Audiobook)

Printed in the U.S.A.

Book design by DesignForBooks.com

Dedication

This book is dedicated to every young man who has ever heard me speak in person. The ones who . . .

- weren't afraid to speak their truth during our classroom discussions;
- stayed after class to share their heart and powerful stories with me privately; and
- wrote the anonymous letters scattered throughout the pages of this book.

Without them, this book would not have been possible.

To those young men, I say, "Thank you for your honesty and transparency. And thank you for sowing a seed that will benefit young men for years to come."

This book is also dedicated to every young man reading it. And I hope you will . . .

- see it's written from the heart of someone who cares;
- understand you have the power to shape your future with the choices you make today; and

- allow the wisdom in this book to propel you to become all you were destined to be.

Finally, I dedicate this book to my amazing mother, Lillie Brewton, who passed away before I published this book. She modeled a life of service and selflessness that continues to fuel my passion for making a positive impact in the lives of teens.

Contents

WHY TEEN GUYS ABSTAIN FROM SEX

1. They know their value   9
2. To be protectors and not predators   15
3. They have discipline and self-control   21
4. They love and respect women   29
5. To be role models for younger sisters   37
6. To protect their future children   43
7. To protect their future spouses   49
8. To avoid negative consequences   57
9. They have dreams and goals   63
10. They are proud of who they are and their decisions   71

WHY TEEN GUYS HAVE SEX

1. They let their hormones control them   77
2. To relieve stress   83
3. Their friends have sex and they feel pressure to fit in   89
4. To brag to their friends   95

5. They face pressure from their fathers and/or other adult men   101
6. To satisfy curiosity   105
7. To gain manhood   109
8. The girls offer sex   113
9. To experience physical pleasure   117
10. They are embarrassed about being a virgin   123

Introduction

Whether you picked this book up on your own, or someone purchased it for you, and you are reading it reluctantly, you are about to learn the truth about sex that many adult men wish they had learned when they were teens. And you will not learn it only from me. Instead, you will mainly gain insights from teen guys like yourself.

How do I know about guys and teen sex?

You may be wondering, How does this woman know anything about guys or teen sex?

Well, let me introduce myself. My name is Jackie Brewton, and I am a youth motivational speaker, health educator and teen relationship expert. I have gained this "inside scoop" from twenty years of experience listening to young men get real (and sometimes even raw) about sex, love, and relationships during my classroom presentations in high schools. They have also written me thousands of letters over the years, sharing their feelings and revealing their choices.

Why am I writing to guys?

I wrote my first book for teen girls. And whenever I read excerpts from that book in my high school classes, guys ask, "Where is our book?"

When I host workshops for teen girls, parents say, "Do you ever do anything for guys? My son needs to hear this message."

After receiving these comments from teen guys and parents for years, I finally recognized how great the need was and realized I was in a perfect position to fill the need. Why? Because there are few people who have had the number of conversations I have had with teen guys about sex or received the number of letters from them on the topic. Conversations and letters too transparent and too good not to share.

How do teen guys respond?

I also wrote this book because of the response I have received from guys in my classes who have written me letters. Like the following . . .

You answered all the questions that I wasn't sure who to ask. Because of you, I look forward to protecting my future wife, my future life and my future marriage.
— **High School Sophomore**

In my personal opinion, your lesson was one of the realest, no <u>the</u> realest lesson I've had in my four years of high school. I've had a few lessons like the one you brought to us, but yours was the entire truth . . . I believe you helped save my life and my girlfriend's.

— High School Senior

I really, really appreciate all you said. I've always had questions and I didn't know where to turn to receive answers. It made everything so much easier the way you came in and let things be known . . . I hugged you when I left. That put the icing on the cake. I could really see in your eyes that everything you were saying was genuine and you have a true passion for helping people. I wish we could speak again on a one-on-one basis.

— High School Junior

With responses like those, why wouldn't I want to reach teen guys without the opportunity to sit in one of my presentations?

And I hope you will appreciate the truth spread throughout these pages as much as the young men who heard me speak in person.

Why is this book necessary?

It breaks my heart to read letter after letter from teen guys who had sex. Many believed it was what they were supposed to do, even if it was not what they wanted to do.

I smile whenever guys stay after class to thank me for removing their pressure to have sex. Of course, some regret their decision to have sex in the past, while others are virgins ashamed of their status. However, a weight is lifted from their shoulders either way when they learn that sex should not define them.

> *I'm a virgin, but my friends all assume I've had sex, so I let them think what they want.*
> *But whenever the subject comes up, I just keep to myself. I just don't want them to think I haven't had sex because I don't want to deal with all the questions that they will ask me.*
> *At the end of the day, I know I'm doing the right thing and I would just like to thank you for reassuring my*

confidence I have in my decision.
— **High School Junior**

When pre-teen and teen guys are encouraged to have sex and made to believe it is a rite of passage into manhood, you need to have information that will help you recognize what you stand to lose or gain when making your own choice.

What will you learn?

Throughout the book, I will share stories of my discussions and interactions with guys and girls. You will also read excerpts from over fifty of the letters I have received.

The book contains two sections. The first includes ten reasons teen guys have told me they abstained from sex. The second includes ten reasons they told me they had sex.

Each chapter is short and includes quotes from teen guys who have participated in my class. I also share my thoughts about each reason guys chose to have sex or abstain. Each chapter ends with five self-reflection questions.

I am most excited about the 100 self-reflection questions in the book. They allow you to take the information you gained reading the book and apply it to your own life.

Despite what popular culture would have you believe, there is no hurry for you to have sex! You can and should wait.

But do not take my word for it. Instead, read for yourself what guys your age had to say about why they did or did not wait and their outcome.

I always tell students they do not have to make ALL the mistakes themselves. And let's be real, with love, sex and relationships, there are plenty of mistakes to be made. So why not learn from others? The good and the bad.

That is what this book is about: helping you learn from other teen guys' decisions about sex so you can experience the relief and bypass the regrets.

The choice is up to you!

WHY TEEN GUYS ABSTAIN FROM SEX

#1

They know their value

I understand the importance of sex and how serious it can be. Even though I'm a guy, you taught me how much value and respect I should have for myself.

— **High School Sophomore**

I interviewed a recent high school graduate once. He told me he hated the double standard fathers often have about sex for their teen sons and daughters. His father would drive him to girls' houses to have sex. And the only thing his father ever told him about sex was that he should always use a condom. However, his father always told his sister she should not have sex because she needed to know her value and worth.

Guys Have Value Too

This young man said, "Boys have value too. But no one ever talks to us about knowing our value when it comes to sex. As an 18-year-old, I wish I was still a virgin. I started having sex in the 9th grade and got a girl pregnant in the 11th grade. I convinced her to have an abortion because I did not want a baby to affect my chances of playing football in college. Now, every time I hear a baby cry, it messes with my head because of the abortion. If my father had given me the same message he gave my sister, I think I would still be a virgin."

You know what? He is right!

The lives, health and futures of boys are as valuable as those of girls. And guys should understand this and treat themselves the way they deserve.

> *I used to think that sex was something a male should achieve and boast about. Now I realize I have value and I shouldn't give my virginity away.*
> **— High School Freshman**

I recently watched a video of a 42-year-old man who made a public vow to abstain from sex until he got married. He wrote this to his future wife while making his vow: You are worth the wait. And I finally believe I am worth the wait too.

He said writing those words reminded him of an experience he had at 19 years old. This experience caused him to believe he was not worth the wait for 23 years.

Although he already had a son, at 19, he vowed to himself and God he would wait until marriage to have sex again. But, unfortunately, when he told his new girlfriend, a virgin, he wanted to wait, she did not share his commitment. And she continued pressuring him to have sex.

She told him, "If you wait until marriage to have sex, you are getting something no one has ever had. But I am getting something everybody has had."

To her, what she was giving him was more valuable than what he would be giving her.

Unfortunately, her words caused him to also believe he did not have value. So he had sex with her, then cheated on her a month later.

It took 23 years before he could confidently say, "I finally believe I am worth the wait."

He later told her how much her statement hurt him. He explained how he would give her something no other woman had ever received—his commitment to wait until marriage to have sex. While she was worried about other girls having his penis, he was prepared to give her something much greater—his promise.

Do not allow decisions from your past to rob you of your sense of worth today.

Let this 42-year-old's story be a cautionary tale for you: Do not allow decisions from your past to rob you of your sense of worth today. Your value is NOT based on your past choices.

You are worth the wait, too. No matter what your peers, the media, older men, and/or girls may tell you otherwise.

> *When I was 14, I lost my virginity to a girl that I didn't date or even know for longer than a month. It wasn't because someone forced me. It was because all my cousins are older than me and they are all sexually active, so I felt as if I should lose my virginity too. It was a mistake. I didn't feel valuable afterwards. After I told my cousins, I was praised; but if I could go back, I would've never lost my virginity to her. All this would have never happened if my cousins were taught their value and if I was taught my value.*
>
> **— High School Senior**

Self-Reflection Questions

1 When you have children, do you plan to have the same expectations for your son and your daughter about their sexual decisions? If not, why?

2 Why do you think parents do not teach guys about their value the same way they teach girls?

3 What other double standard(s) bother you about how guys and girls are taught and/or treated with sex? Why?

4 Do you think your choices/behavior would be any different if you thought about your value before making your decisions? If so, how?

5 What difference would it make in our culture/society if we taught guys they have value?

#2

To be protectors and not predators

Being a 'jock', most of the stuff you said I just sort of thought, Yeah, yeah, statistics can make anything look bad or vice versa. But when you got to the part about being the protector, and not the predator . . . that got to me. Having two sisters myself, I know how it feels to protect. I like it. Before I wanted to just have sex, but I now know that makes me a predator. I have reevaluated my view on sex because of your talk.

— **High School Junior**

A predator is someone who takes advantage of the vulnerability of another person for his/her own selfish gain. A protector keeps others safe from harm.

Some guys are aware there are underlying reasons girls have sex that have nothing to do with them, while others are oblivious to this. If you are one of the guys who does not have a clue, let me share a few reasons girls may have sex that have nothing to do with you: daddy issues, low self-esteem, and even prior rape or sexual molestation.

It is very important to note here; I am not saying all girls are helpless and only have sex because they are broken. But, these are a few examples I see far too often.

Are You A Predator or Protector?

Some guys (not all, but some), will take advantage of girls' vulnerability to get sex. And that is a predator.

I am not saying every sexually active guy is a predator. Some guys do not know if a girl has these underlying struggles. And some girls have no issues. But when a young lady has sex, she is not protecting herself from the physical and emotional pain that so often accompanies sex. And neither is her partner.

Like the one quoted above, young men who understand this will not risk their health or their partner's. But they will step up and protect themselves and young women from any potential harm.

During the whole time you were speaking, I had my girlfriend's emotions and future in mind, and how I wanted

*her to succeed in life so she can better herself. You made me realize that she doesn't deserve to have a boy make her emotionally unstable. Instead, she deserves a boy that will do what is best for her so she can push forward in life.
You have inspired me to be a better young man for her.*

— **High School Senior**

Be A Man You Can Be Proud Of

One of my mentees, who had sex at 14, stopped having sex at 23. I met him when he was 25. I thought his story was powerful. So, I asked him if I could videotape him sharing his story during an interview.

Several things led to his decision to stop having sex, but I will discuss one of them right now.

One reason he stopped having sex was that he knew many women he had sex with were medicating pain. They dealt with low self-esteem, absent fathers, previous rape/molestation, etc.

He felt like a drug dealer. Giving those broken women more hits or doses, which was keeping them the same or making them worse.

He realized he had become a predator, which was something he was not proud of.

When my mentee was a teenager, he may not have regretted how he treated girls. But something happens when you grow up and become a man. You can see the negative effects your past choices may have had on not only your life but the other person's as well.

A father who sat in on a session once approached me afterward to share the following:

> *I am rarely emotional. But tears came to my eyes as I listened to your stories. It broke my heart to hear why teen girls have sex and how devastated they often are because of sex. I had flashbacks to how I was when I was a teenager. I wondered how many girls I may have hurt back then may still be broken today. It is not something I am proud of. And now that I have a teenage daughter, I pray that she never dates a guy like I was when I was a teenager.*

I hope you will live long enough to be an adult man one day. At which time you must do the same thing this man did, remember your past. What will those memories be? Will they be memories you will be proud of?

Or will you also have regrets about the sexual choices you made when you were a teenager? Will you have a daughter and fear you may have to reap what you have sown?

To be honest, I'm one of those guys who refuses sex when my girlfriend asks because I want her to know that I respect her. I have extremely high expectations for her, even if she doesn't. Because she means the world to me, I want to protect her and love her for the right reasons instead of all the wrong. Even though it does get really tempting to just go ahead and be like any other boy and have sex frequently, I want to be different because I respect my girlfriend a lot.

— High School Senior

Self-Reflection Questions

1 Were you aware that the reasons teen girls have sex may differ from the reasons teen guys have sex? If not, why do you think you were not aware?

2 Does being a protector resonate with you? If so, how?

3 When you become an adult, which do you think you will be most proud of? Being a protector or predator?

4 Are there any decisions you have made that you think could come back to haunt you if you have a daughter one day? If so, what?

5 What can you do now to make sure you will be proud later of the choices you are making?

#3

They have discipline and self-control

No matter how tempting and life-changing sex could be, a real man knows how to have self-control.

— **High School Junior**

Sex is one of the most difficult areas for teen guys to show self-control because of their hormones. But teenagers who can control their hormones are teenagers who have a great chance of succeeding.

If you can control your body, everything else will be easy in comparison.

If you can control your body, everything else will be easy in comparison. And you will always need to have self-control.

Many addictions we struggle with in our country are due to self-control failures (i.e., alcoholism, gambling, excessive shopping/spending, over-eating, drugs, sex, pornography, etc.).

The only way to develop self-control is to practice. And with sex—you are practicing saying YES or you are practicing saying NO. The choice is yours!

The Self-Control Struggle is Real

I will not sugar coat it—if you practice self-control, you will need a lot of discipline.

noun: self-discipline

*correction or regulation of oneself
for the sake of improvement*

Self-Discipline is essential in life, yet it is often one of the least developed skills for teens and adults alike. It will prevent you from destructive behaviors such as over-eating, over-spending, and cheating on your spouse.

Which reminds me of the story of my two good friends, Tony and Julie. When they met, they were both twenty-four years old. Julie was a virgin and Tony was not.

Check out the conversation I had with Tony to see how he handled self-control while dating Julie:

Tony: When we started dating, Julie told me she was a virgin. She also said she would not have sex

#3 They have discipline & self-control

with me or anyone else until her wedding night.

Me: I love that she knew her value. So, she basically said, 'This is my price. You can either pay this price or you can keep stepping, and I will wait for someone who will.' I wish more girls were this confident.

Tony: Had I met her in high school or college, that is what I would have done—kept stepping. At that time, I was not looking for 'Mrs. Right.' I was looking for 'Ms. Right Now.' But at twenty-four years old, knowing she was a virgin was very attractive. Her value in my eyes went up. *[Anything that is rare is automatically worth more.]* We dated for a year before we got engaged. And we were engaged for a year. We had sex for the first time on our wedding night.

Me: Wow. Most girls think no guy would wait, especially not two years.

Tony: I am glad Julie raised the standard and required me to marry her before having sex. She showed me how much self-control I had while we were dating. And that self-control keeps me from cheating on her now that we are married. *[And they have been happily married for 30 years now and counting].* I have more women hitting on me with a ring on my finger than I ever did without.

Me: Oh, my goodness. That is what I tell the students—you do not get discipline and self-control as a wedding gift. If you do not have self-control before you get married, saying two words—"I Do"—will not give you the self-control you will need to stay faithful to your spouse.

Discipline is the key to success.

Discipline is the key to success. If you can show self-control in the key area of sex, it will pay huge dividends in every other area of your life.

This area will be the most difficult for you to have discipline because it is a natural desire. But, if you have discipline with sex, the sky is the limit on how successful you will be in life. This is because you will have mastered the most difficult thing in your life . . . yourself.

I spoke with Tony again, and he provided more information about his decision.

Tony: Here is something else you can share with your students. Abstaining from sex is a great way to determine how strong you are. I had no idea I was that strong. If a buddy had told me a month before I met Julie that I would ever go two years without sex, I would have told him he was crazy. I will always appreciate Julie for helping me see my true strength.

How Strong are You?

Some people will never know their true strength because they do not challenge themselves. It is easy to say you have the discipline and self-control to abstain from sex. The only way to prove it is with your actions.

A sexually active sixteen-year-old guy once told me, "I could stop having sex if I wanted to. It is not that I do not have self-control. I just like it. But if I wanted to stop, I could."

I said, "Who are you trying to convince—me or you? If you really have the self-control it takes to abstain from sex, prove it! Not to me. Prove it to yourself. Because until you stop having sex, those are words anyone can say."

Now it is your turn.

If you are having sex but feel as if you can stop at any time like the young man above, prove it to yourself and accept this challenge:

Some people will never know their true strength because they do not challenge themselves.

Stop having sex for at least 30 days.

If that is not a problem for you, see how long you can go without it. If you cannot do it or it is difficult, know that you need to work harder to develop this self-discipline skill.

> *I am a virgin. I expect the best for myself, and believe the self-control I have upheld with regards to athletics and academics spills over to other parts of my life. When*

other people at my age give in to sex, I see physical and emotional pain. When I think about giving in to sex, I only see heartbreak, disappointment and one more unneeded weight on my shoulders. I learned that no matter how tempting and life changing sex can be, a real man knows how to have self-control.

— **High School Junior**

Self-Reflection Questions

1 Can you think of any celebrities or athletes who allowed a lack of self-control to have a negative impact on their career or life? If so, who & how?

2 Are there any areas where you show discipline/self-control? What helps you to do it successfully?

3 What areas in your life are you not demonstrating discipline/self-control? What prevents you from practicing self-control?

4 What is one area where you are not practicing self-control, but you are willing to put forth an effort to practice self-control?

5 What are 1–3 things you can do for it to be easier to reach your goal?

#4

They love and respect women

To be honest, I'm one of those guys who refuses sex when my girlfriend asks because I want her to know that I respect her. Because she means the world to me, I want to protect her and love her for the right reasons instead of all the wrong.

— **High School Senior**

When you love and respect the person you are in a relationship with, you will do what is best for her. You will also do everything in your power to NOT cause her harm.

Sex is never the best choice for teens to make due to all the risks. So, having sex is not how to show her you love her. Abstaining from sex is.

You know who else thinks sex is not the best choice for teens? Students. Even the ones having sex.

They agree that teenage sex is never the best way to become successful or reach their dreams and goals.

When I ask them when they believe it would be a wise time for two people in a relationship to have sex, I get a broad range of answers. The one I normally focus on (and it typically comes from a girl) is, "When you are in love."

Sex ≠ Love

Which brings me to the next question: How can you tell when you love someone?

The most important part of love is the selfless nature of love.

Their responses are often superficial—It's a feeling you can't explain. You can't stop thinking about them. You get butterflies in your stomach when you see them, etc.

I explain to them those things are called "chemistry," which is a part of love. But it is not the most important part.

The most important part of love is the selfless nature of love. Where you will always do what is best for them and you would do nothing to hurt them. And students agree with that definition.

I then pose this question to the class, "If the following two things are true:

1. It is never the best choice for teens to have sex.

2. When you love someone, you will always do what is best for them.

Then, is it ever possible for teenagers to have sex and truly love each other?"

I will often get this push back from a guy: "But what if you did not pressure her to have sex. What if it was her idea? Why should I feel bad about having sex with a girl that I did not pressure?"

To which I will respond, "If you truly love her, I do not care if she comes to you and offers you sex. You would say to her, "Baby, I promise I am not cheating on you, but I am going to do what is best for you even when you will not do what is best for yourself."

And that is what I shared with a young man named Josh whose girlfriend Shelby wanted me to talk to him.

Shelby: Please tell my boyfriend what you told us in class about guys' inability to get tested for HPV (human papilloma virus).

Me: She is right. There is not a test for males to determine whether they have the type of HPV that could cause cervical cancer in females. However, they will know they have the virus if one of their partners tests positive for the virus.

Shelby: We have been having sex for three months. His ex-girlfriend and I are friends, and I know that she has HPV because she told me. I want

Josh to understand why I want to stop having sex. I do not want to put myself at risk of getting HPV any more than I already have.

Josh to Shelby: How do you know she didn't get the STD from someone she had sex with after we broke up? She might not have had it while we were dating.

Me to Josh: That is possible, but it is also possible that she had it while you were dating.

Me to Shelby: How old are you?

Shelby: Seventeen.

Me to Josh: Let me ask you a question. If you had a seventeen-year-old daughter or little sister, would you want her to have sex at that age?

Josh: No!

Me: Why?

Josh: Because of the consequences.

Me: Is that because you would love her too much to see her risk getting the consequences that may come with that decision?

Josh: Exactly!

Me: Why can't you love Shelby that much?

Josh: I do love her! I have never pressured her to have sex.

Me: Do you know what you should do if you loved her? Even if she pressured you to have sex, you would not do it because you would do what is best for her even when she would not do what is best for herself.

Put Her Best Interests Above Your Sex Interests

How can this young man stand in front of his girlfriend and say he would not want his own daughter or little sister doing what he is asking her to do?

Real love always does what is best for the other person. If Josh did not think that sex would be the best choice for his daughter or little sister, he should have loved Shelby enough to not let her make the same poor choice.

Also, when you love someone, you try to help her become the best person she can be and encourage her to reach her goals. For example, if she tells you she does not want to have sex and you claim to love her, you will not try to talk her out of her goal.

Instead, you would respect her decisions and do everything in your power to help her achieve her goals.

You would also avoid situations that could cause her to compromise her standards. Even when she may be willing to give in and have sex, you would not let her. Because you would value and respect her like the young man mentioned in the letter below.

> *Two years ago, I met the love of my life, and you may think that it was just teen love, but it wasn't like that at all. Because I loved him so much, I told him that I'd be willing to lose my virginity to him. When we were alone in his house, I told him that I wanted to have sex with him. His reply shocked me. He told me that as much as he'd love to have sex with me, he would never want me to break the promise that I made to myself. He told me that he loves me too much to hurt me. We are still together, and it's almost our two-year and three-month anniversary, and I love him more than ever. During your visit with us, I fell in love with him more. I love the fact that I'm still a virgin, which wouldn't have happened if it weren't for him saying no.*
>
> **— High School Senior Girl**

Now that is real love!

Self-Reflection Questions

1 What does respect look like to you in a relationship?

2 In a relationship, do you believe that respect should be earned or given freely? Why?

3 Have you ever shown someone respect even when they did not respect themselves? If so, how did it make you feel?

4 Have you ever seen selfless love in a relationship where one gives up what they want to benefit the other? If so, who was it and how did they show selfless love?

5 Have you ever demonstrated selfless love in a relationship? If so, how?

#5

To be role models for younger sisters

I have to be a good example for my little sister because I don't want her to be mistreated by other guys. If she were to get hurt thinking that it's okay because her brother used to have sex with girls, I would be devastated. No, that's not gonna happen, which is why I'm still a virgin. You made me want to show my little sister that there are men out there who aren't looking for sex.

— **High School Junior**

After finishing a presentation to a health class of high school juniors and seniors one day, five young men stayed after class to speak with me. The last young man who had patiently waited for me to finish speaking with the others only wanted to say, "Thank You!"

I told him how much it meant that he had waited so long to let me know how much he appreciated and benefitted from my presentation.

I also told him I was sure he was already making good decisions even before hearing me speak. He dropped his head and said nothing. I said, "But you will START making good decisions after today, right? Because when you know better, you do better." He smiled and said, "Yes!"

Even though he seemed shy and had little to say, he was not in a hurry to leave. So, I made small talk with him, asking him about his life, grades, etc.

Act Like Your Little Sister's Watching

When I asked him about his home life, he said he lived with his mom and two younger sisters, aged 10 and 13. So, I said to him:

"If you have two younger sisters, I know that you are going to be a great role model for them, right? You will show them how they should expect their boyfriends to treat them when they are older based on how they see you treat your girlfriends.

Do you understand what a huge responsibility it is to know that you could influence your younger sisters' lives to that degree? That is HUGE man! And you know what? I believe you can meet that challenge.

Your decision to treat the girls you date with respect by not having sex with them is SO much bigger than the benefit of abstaining for you personally. This is not only about you. This is also about what you are teaching your younger sisters about men and relationships.

You can show your little sisters what REAL love is. And that is as simple as doing what is best for the person you are dating. It is also about doing nothing that you know could hurt her.

Every time you think about having sex, say to yourself, 'This is not ONLY about me!'

Don't you think that will make it easier to stick to your commitment if you know your decision is NOT only about you?"

He smiled and confidently said, 'YES!" I hugged him, told him I believed in him and he left.

Be Her Role Model

I will ask you the same question I ask the guys in my classes.

Would you want your little sister dating a guy like you? If the answer is no, that is a problem. It means you are not a good role model. Do you know the best way to prevent your little sister from having sex? It is by modeling the behavior you want her to demonstrate and expect from guys.

When you asked whether I would

> *want my sister to date a guy like me, that's when I realized I'm changing the way I act towards females, not just for me but also for my sister. I'm going to lead by example.*
>
> **— High School Junior**

You can tell your little sister all day long that she doesn't have to have sex in a relationship. But, if she knows you are having sex with the young ladies you date, she will likely believe it is what she must do when she gets into a relationship.

A lot of girls have sex because they don't think they have a choice. They believe no guy would date them without sex.

If your sister can see you in relationships without sex, it gives her hope it is possible. She now has a standard to which she can hold all the guys she dates.

> *What you said made me want to be a better man. It made me look back and do a mental check to see if I was being a superior role model for my little sister. I want her to see me and think, 'One day I want a love one in my life who is just like my brother.' You made me want to*

show my little sister that there are men out there who aren't looking for sex.

— **High School Sophomore**

Self-Reflection Questions

1 Have you had any positive role models in your family to show you how to be a role model for others? If so, who is it and what did they model for you?

2 Do you know of any positive well-known role models for teens with relationships? Who? What makes them a role model?

3 Based on how you treat girls in relationships, would you want your little sister or future daughter to date a guy like you? Why or why not?

4 Who do you feel a responsibility to be a positive role model for and why?

5 How does it make you feel to know that your choices can affect others' choices in a negative or positive way?

#6

To protect their future children

I've gotten closer and closer to losing my virginity until you came to speak to us. You gave me a whole other perspective. You made me think about my kids, about how I want them to live, about the kind of parents they'll have. I think every day about the type of father I'd be. Hearing everything you had to say makes me want to keep their future safe. As you said, 'One day my family will be the most important thing in my life, so why wouldn't my future family be a priority right now?'

— **High School Freshman**

Most teens agree they want their kids to have better lives than they have. So when you choose to be a protector rather than a predator, it means not only protecting your girlfriend. It also includes protecting your future children from less-than-ideal circumstances.

Protecting future children sounds wonderful. But, unfortunately, many teens do not realize their choices as teenagers have everything to do with giving their kids that better life.

Do you know what I have seen over the years? Teens sometimes behave as if something magical will happen when they become an adult, putting them in position to be an excellent parent and give their children a perfect life.

They do not always understand that their decisions while they are teens will determine the lifestyle their children will have.

Will Your Children Pay for Your Decisions?

I asked the students in a class once how many wanted to get married. About 80% of the students raised their hands.

I then asked them, "Why do you want to get married?"

The first person to respond was a very vocal young man bragging about how much sex he had.

Check out our conversation below:

Young Man: So, I can have kids.

Me: You don't have to be married to have kids. People have kids every day without being married.

Young Man: Nah, I want to be there for my kids. I won't desert my kids as my father did. I will be in the house with my kids every day.

A few other guys chimed in and echoed what he said. They also wanted to be 'better men than their fathers' and be in the house with their kids.

Me: So, what you are saying is not that you want to get married to have kids. You want to get married to do what is best for your kids?

Young Man: Yeah, that's it. I am getting married so I can do what is best for my kids.

Me: So, does that mean you will stop having sex as a teenager?

Young Man: Now, I did not say all of that!

Me: Then you lied. Because you said what you thought would be best for your kids was for their father to be in the house with them every day. Yet, you are having sex as a teenager, which means you could get the girl pregnant. The condom could break this weekend, which happens all the time. If you become a father at 16, I am not sure you can be in the house with your kids every day like you said you wanted to be.

It sounds honorable to say you want to do what is best for your future kids. But do your daily decisions reflect that desire? Do you want it bad enough to make the choices you need to make now to give them that best life?

And I will say the same thing to you—when deciding whether to have sex or not, think about what would happen if a pregnancy occurred. Then ask yourself whether you would have made the best choice for your child.

Having sex before you can give your child the life you want them to have is risking their best life for your temporary pleasure. As my friend's father used to say, "Never gamble what you cannot afford to lose!"

What would a selfless protector do?

After hearing you speak about remaining abstinent, my entire perspective on sex has changed. Over and over we, as teenagers, hear how having sex before marriage can change our lives; but you were the first person to explain how it can impact others. All my life, my entire mindset behind involvement with girls was to be as different from my dad as I could. You helped me to realize that my behavior now is potentially changing not only my own, but my future child's future. I finally understand that I'm risking my kid growing up the same way I did. I want a bright future for my kids and if that means no sex, then no sex it shall be. I know this will be difficult because no sooner had I made this decision than was a temptation revealed. But your words and my own past remind me of my goal and to keep my focus on reaching it.

— High School Senior

Self-Reflection Questions:

1 Do you want to get married and have children? Why or why not?

2 Do you want your kids to have a better life than you have? Why or why not?

3 Have you thought about the life you would want your future children to have? If so, what will that life look like?

   a. What kind of school will they attend?

   b. What kind of neighborhood/house will they live in?

   c. What type of extracurricular activities will they participate in?

4 Are the choices you are making now putting you in a position to give your future children the life you described? If so, how? If not, why not?

5 What are three things you can do during your teen years to ensure you provide the best life for your future children?

#7

To protect their future spouses

Your call to action, that a real man would do what is best for his partner no matter his personal desires, has motivated me and prompted me to uphold that fact. I strive to be that man that you described, one that a girl would be happy to have. A real man makes decisions that makes his life better and has the courage to say no. You have definitely influenced me to wait to have sex until marriage so, I will be able to step up as a man to provide for my future family.

— **High School Junior**

A real man protects and provides for his family. Do not wait until you meet your future wife to begin protecting her. The best way to protect your future wife is by giving her the best and "freest" husband possible when you meet her—one who is not bound by disease and other baggage from past relationships.

Your Future Starts Now!

Let's say you have sex as a teenager and continue having sex during your college years. Because you are doing what society says men should do. At 25, you decide you are ready to settle down and have a wife and kids. You fall in love with and marry a virgin. A year after you get married, your wife goes to the gynecologist for her annual pelvic exam. Her pap smear comes back abnormal. They do a follow-up test and it shows she has HPV, the type that causes cervical cancer.

She goes through the following treatment plan . . .

First, they scrape your wife's cervix to remove all the pre-cancer cells. Then, she has to return every three months for a follow-up. If they see pre-cancerous cells on any of her follow up visits, they will remove a portion of her cervix. The cervix keeps the baby in the uterus when a woman gets pregnant. So, if they remove a portion of her cervix, she will have difficulty carrying a baby full term. And she will be prone to miscarriages.

If they discover pre-cancerous cells on any of your wife's future three-month visits, they may have to perform a hysterectomy. Which means they remove her uterus and she can never have children.

How will you feel about yourself as a man when you have to watch your wife pay for your past?

If real men protect and provide for their families, then being a real man starts right now!

Choose to abstain from any activities that could put your future spouse at risk. And be the man who always does what is best for those he loves and will love one day.

> *I am now determined to remain abstinent until marriage. I do plan on marrying a virgin because I have high expectations of my future wife. I don't want to settle. And I hope she has equally high expectations of me. I now realize that just because she's not right here right now, doesn't mean I shouldn't act like it. My view of staying a virgin is not because I'm not ready to have sex or that I'm scared, I would just like for my future wife to have all of me and not pieces of me that previous women left.*
>
> **— High School Sophomore**

I will never forget a conversation I had with a young man in class one day. He said there was a girl he liked a lot and could even see a long-term future with her. There was only one problem . . . she was a virgin and did not want to have sex until she got married.

Although he respected her more for her decision, he was not ready to give up sex and be faithful to one person.

His solution? To "put her on the shelf" until he was ready to settle down and be faithful.

He needed to be brought back down to earth, so I challenged him to consider:

> How can you be sure this young lady will wait for you until you tire of having sex with other girls?
>
> How much do you really care about this young lady if you will put her at risk of contracting an STD from you after you have finished "sowing your wild oats?"
>
> Let's talk about how your plan could play out:
>
> You love and respect your girlfriend enough not to have sex with her. And you plan to settle down with her once you finish having as much sex as you want with girls you do not care about.
>
> While having sex with these other young ladies, you contract an STD, maybe even HPV, which you cannot get tested for.

#7 To protect their future spouses

> *After you settle down, you reconnect with the girlfriend you have "loved" all along. Then, the two of you get married and you give her an STD you contracted while you were "sexing it up" during your teen years.*
>
> *If love is about protecting the person you claim to love, do you feel you protected her?*

Afterward, he realized how unfair his so-called "solution" was to the young lady he claimed to see a future with.

And I hope his story helps you realize what is at stake when you have sex as a teen.

It is not about you having as much "fun" as you can while you are young.

It is about deciding now, as a teen, what will set you up to have the life you desire for you and your future wife.

> *After realizing the reality and seriousness behind sex I have taken a vow of abstinence until marriage and will take it serious. I couldn't imagine what my life would be like if my girlfriend got pregnant or if I gave her an STD. I would be completely distraught. So, I am choosing to pay now by being dedicated to becoming the man I know I can be*

so that when I become that man I can give my wife the life she deserves.

— **High School Senior**

Self-Reflection Questions

1 Have you thought about the type of woman you would want to marry one day? What would you like her to be like? (Think about her emotional AND physical attributes).

2 A lot of guys say they plan to marry a virgin so they do not have to worry about dealing with physical and emotional baggage from their future wife's past relationships. Is that what you plan to do as well? Why or why not?

3 How would you feel if you were not a virgin when you got married, but your wife was; and she contracted an STD from you after getting married you did not even know you had?

4 What would it mean to you if your future wife was intentionally making choices during her dating years to protect you and your marriage even before she meets you?

5 What choices can you make now to ensure that you are protecting your future wife even before you meet her?

#8

To avoid negative consequences

Thank you for confirming that I have made the correct choice in choosing to be a virgin. I am a guy and it's really hard to fight the urges, but I have paid attention to what is happening around me (STDs and teenage pregnancy). I don't want those things to be a part of my life. I am a football player and I have a few schools looking at me so I may have a future. I don't want to risk messing that up.

— High School Senior

While fear is not the best motivator for avoiding sex, for some young men it is all the motivation they need. These are the young men who will learn from others' mistakes and do not insist on making their own.

They recognize they are not invincible and STDs do not discriminate. STDs don't care how good of an athlete you are, how good looking you are or how good looking your partner is. They are a by-product of the act . . . and can still happen even if you "wrap it up."

With that knowledge, smart young men realize that negative consequences are a legitimate risk. So they abstain because they are not willing to take the chance.

Risky Business

The guys who do not mind taking that chance will say that bad things do not happen every time you have sex. And they never think it will happen to them. But remember this:

It may not happen every time, but it can happen any time and all it takes is one time.

A 16-year-old guy approached me one Friday after class because he was afraid he may have an STD. He had been experiencing some symptoms of one of the STDs I discussed in class.

He only had sex one time with a young lady he was not in a relationship with. And he wanted to know where he could get tested without his parents

#8 To avoid negative consequences 59

discovering. He believed they would kill him if they knew he had sex.

I texted the young man the phone number for the local health department. I realized later it was a mistake for him to have my cell phone number. Why? Because he texted or called me at least ten times over that weekend. He was in a panic because by the time he reached his older brother to take him to the doctor, the office was closed. And it would not open again until Tuesday (Monday was a holiday).

Every time he contacted me over the weekend, his symptoms had gotten worse. I believed at least some of what he described was in his head. His fears were so exaggerated it was almost humorous.

To make a long story short, he eventually told his dad. They went to the doctor Tuesday and he was diagnosed with gonorrhea. Remember, this was his <u>one, and only, time having sex</u>.

When I spoke with him afterwards, I told him he was fortunate the STD he contracted was curable. It could have been much worse.

I asked him if the pleasure he experienced from sex was worth the stress he had experienced over those four days.

His response?

"Absolutely not! I regret ever having sex!"

Which reminds me of a quote by Jim Rohn:

"We must all suffer from one of two pains: the pain of discipline or the pain of regret.

The difference is discipline weighs ounces while regret weighs tons."

This young man suffered from the second pain, because he could not handle the struggle that comes with the first.

It is up to you to decide which you prefer.

Thanks to your knowledge and how you gave it to our class, I now have a new quote to think about which will help me with my decisions for the rest of my life. 'It won't happen EVERY time, but it can happen ANY time and it only takes ONE time.' I'm happy to inform you that I have now chosen NO times. Thank you for your investment in my future.
I won't let you or my generation down.

— **High School Junior**

Self-Reflection Questions

1 Is fear enough to motivate you to abstain from sex? Why or why not?

2 Can you think of any teen guy who had sex and had to deal with a negative consequence as a result? What was the consequence? And how did he handle it?

3 Have you thought about how your life would change if you became a teen dad?

    a. How will your parents feel when you tell them?

    b. How will you provide for your child while trying to finish high school?

    c. How will it impact your ability to continue your schooling beyond high school?

4 If you contract an STD, how will you pay to get treated? If it is an incurable STD, how will you tell future partners you are infected?

5 Have you thought about the potential legal consequences? What if the young lady you have sex with says afterwards that it was not consensual? How would you feel going through the legal process of defending yourself?

#9

They have dreams and goals

I'm not trying to let a girl come and take my dreams away. Like you said, pay now and play later; and that's what I am going to do. I am not ready to throw away my chance at a bright future for a little temporary pleasure.

— High School Sophomore

This young man has his priorities in order. He has dreams and goals he wants to achieve. He also knows sex will always be there after he has achieved them. He has discovered the ultimate goals he wants so badly that he will not let anyone or anything prevent him from reaching them.

I call it his "Yes."

*There have been times where I could
have had sex, but chose not to because
I had a bigger yes, a bigger dream
and a vision for my future.*

— **High School Junior**

Just Say "Yes!"

One day a young man asked if he and his girlfriend could speak with me after class. He shared:

"My girlfriend heard you speak in her health class in March and was pregnant at the time. She had a miscarriage shortly after your presentation. We were 'lucky' that we did not have to deal with the consequence of the pregnancy. After hearing you speak, my girlfriend told me she wanted to stop having sex. I was not in agreement and continued to pressure her for sex.

She kept telling me I would understand why she wanted to stop if I could hear you speak. And she was excited when she found out you would be returning to speak to my health class too. After hearing you yesterday, I GOT IT! I totally understand why we should stop having sex and I told her I would not pressure her for sex anymore. I have always had a dream of playing football at the University of Georgia and that is what I am going to use as my 'Yes'.

He then said, "Getting to play football at UGA will be my motivation to keep me away from sex. I don't want to risk getting that opportunity."

Having a "Yes" in your life is important because it gives you a goal beyond temporary pleasure. Physical pleasure is one of the worst reasons for you to have sex because it gives you a false, fleeting version of actual fulfillment.

Your "Yes" is the real thing, the true satisfaction you desire in life. If you know what your bigger "Yes" is, you will not be tempted by short-term distractions like sex that could keep you from realizing those dreams.

> *I'm a virgin and have been proud of that. Since my freshman year, people have always acted like being a virgin is a bad thing and some of my old friends laughed at me for being one. But I actually didn't care about what people said because people nowadays make a lot of dumb decisions because they want to 'fit in.' I choose not to 'fit in' with the crowd and be a leader and not fall into temptation but actually be man enough to fight it until I'm married to the right woman in my life.*
>
> **— High School Senior**

Consider the Risks vs. the Rewards

Several years ago, I worked with a program that sponsored an after-school leadership club in several area high schools. A senior star basketball player came to the meeting one day. He was with a young lady who attended the meetings regularly. The young lady went inside the room where the meeting would take place, while the young man stood in the hall. I talked with him since I had never seen him at the meeting before.

Here is how our conversation went:

Me: Is that your girlfriend you came to the meeting with today?

Basketball Player: No, I don't do relationships—too much drama. I am focused on my basketball. A girlfriend would be a distraction.

Me: That makes perfect sense. Well, do you do sex?

Basketball Player: Yeah, I do sex. I just don't do relationships.

Me: Well, don't you know that sex also brings drama?

Basketball Player: Yeah, but that is some drama I am willing to deal with.

Me: Are you having sex with the young lady you came to the meeting with today?

Basketball Player: Yeah, we are having sex.

As we continued to talk, I discovered he was also having sex with other young ladies at his school.

Me: How can you feel good about yourself as a young man when taking advantage of these young ladies like that?

Basketball Player: Look, lady, I don't lie to these girls. I have never told a girl that I love her. They know I don't do relationships and they are not my girlfriend.

I called my friend, Michael, over to speak with him and shared what the basketball player and I had discussed. I then told Michael I asked the young man how he could treat those young ladies that way.

And Michael took over and had this very insightful chat with the young man:

Michael: Man, I don't want to talk with you about what you are doing to the young ladies. I want to talk with you about what you are doing to yourself. I know your reputation. I hear about you all over this county. I know how good you are on the court. I know how much potential you have. I understand why some guys have sex. Because they don't think their lives will amount to anything anyway. So, what if they get an STD? It is not like they were planning to go far in life. So, what if they get a girl pregnant? They will probably bounce like they have seen so many other men do. But, with the future and potential I see ahead of you, I do not understand why you would have sex. That is like you going to Las Vegas to place a million-dollar bet while these other dudes are betting a quarter.

And that is what it boils down to . . . what do you think you are risking? You only consider something an "at-risk" behavior if you think you are risking something. Likewise, you will only try to protect your future if you think you have one.

So, ask yourself this: "Is my future worth risking or saving?

> *When you came to my classroom and spoke, I became more comfortable with myself. I am a teenage male in high school that hasn't had sex by choice. I feel that it is not necessary or even the 'cool' thing to do while in high school, even while friends around me say it's the best. To me, my 'sex' or 'feel good' is accomplishing goals and being something in my future that will later set the foundation for my family and myself. Sex would completely complicate that plan.*
>
> **— High School Junior**

Self-Reflection Questions:

1. Have you determined your "Yes?" If so, what is it?
2. If you have not determined your "Yes," what will be your motivation to prevent you from having sex?
3. Name three goals you want to reach in the next 3–5 years.
4. List at least one thing you can do within the next week to help you reach each goal.
5. List at least one decision you could make that would prevent you from reaching each one of your goals.

#10

They are proud of who they are and their decisions

You showed me that holding myself to a higher standard is much more important than worrying about what people think about me being a virgin.

— High School Sophomore

When you choose to abstain, you do so because you know who you are, what you want, and what it takes to get there. And you are proud of that decision. When you are proud of a choice, you are invested in seeing it through.

Fear can be overcome in several ways.

Young men who are proud of their decision to abstain because they want to make the best choice for their future, will be much more successful in maintaining their commitment than those who abstain because they fear the consequences.

Are You Proud Enough to Wait?

"Pride is a better motivator than fear."
—John Wooden

Today's culture encourages young men to take pride in their virility not virginity. So, many guys do not even consider abstaining from sex a choice worthy of being proud of.

But think about it, what is there to be proud of about having sex as a teen?

It doesn't make you a "real man," or a better husband for your future wife. It isn't an accurate indicator of your value as a young man. It does not make you a respected role model for your little sister.

And having sex as a teen will not help you develop the discipline needed to reach your future goals. It also will not help you establish a lasting legacy you can be proud of sharing with your future children one day.

A young man told me after class one day he was a virgin until he was 17. Then, he was proud of himself for doing something that many teenage boys have not done.

Unfortunately, he gained a new group of friends he allowed to pressure him into having sex. He said he had all these visions in his head about how he would feel after he lost his virginity. He thought he would feel like a man.

He then said, "I will admit that the sex felt good. But the first thought that came to my mind when the sex was over was, 'Dang, now I am like everyone else. I don't have anything left to feel proud of because I did what adults expect all teenagers to do.'"

Be Your Own Man

This young man felt like he had become average. And believe me when I tell you, average is so overrated.

Ordinary people do not get remembered. The people who stand out are the people who follow their own path (not the people who blend in). And that is something to be proud of.

Like John Wooden said, pride is an excellent motivator. Why not take pride in a decision that puts your best interests before your sex interests?

> *The people who stand out are the people who follow their own path (not the people who blend in).*

> *I'm an 18-year-old senior and I am a virgin and proud. I've had 4 girlfriends the whole time I've been in high school . . . Some of my best friends say they wish they were still virgins because you can only [lose] it that one time.*
>
> **— High School Senior**

Self-Reflection Questions

1 Why do you think pride is a better motivator than fear?

2 Are you making decisions you are proud of? If so, what are they? If not, what are they and why aren't you proud of those decisions?

3 Who do you want to be proud of you and your decisions, besides yourself? Peers, friends, parents, siblings, youth leader, etc.?

4 Do you prefer to blend in or follow your own path? Why?

5 Name one decision you have made as a teen that made you feel like everyone else afterwards. What is one thing you can do to combat feeling average and stand out from your peers?

WHY TEEN GUYS HAVE SEX

#1

They let their hormones control them

You have really inspired me to change my sexual habits. I have been sexually active since my freshman year of high school, and I'm a junior now. Sex gradually became a part of me and it got to the point where my hormones controlled my actions. I have made many stupid decisions by letting my hormones control me, but hearing you speak makes me want to take control and save myself from getting stuck in a negative situation that I would have to deal with for the rest of my life.

— **High School Junior**

Some young men will say they cannot control their hormones. But if that is true, all those young men are at risk of becoming inmates one day. Let me explain . . .

Imagine a scenario where a young man has a young lady at his house. One thing leads to the next. And right before he puts on a condom, she changes her mind and tells him she does not want to go any further. If a young man is "incapable" of controlling his hormones (as so many young men believe), one of two things will happen:

1. He will either badger her until he wears her down and she finally gives in even though sex is not what she wants. This is NOT consensual sex.
2. He will force himself on her and rape her.

In either situation, the issue is NOT that the young man is "incapable" of controlling his hormones. He is simply unwilling to.

Boundaries Matter

Sure, it may be more difficult for young men to control their hormones once they are aroused. But why wait until then to control them?

My advice to you? If you stay away from situations that elevate your hormones, you won't have to figure out how to control them after things have started.

This means knowing your boundaries when it comes to how far you will go with a young lady. And staying clear of things like porn that elevate your hormone levels.

If you make it a habit of consuming sexual images via music, movies and/or pornography, you will constantly battle your hormones.

Instead, try limiting your exposure to sexually charged and explicit media. You will most likely find that sex will become "out of sight, out of mind," so to speak.

> *You made me realize that a real man doesn't have to have sex when he is a teenager or whenever to be a man. It's worth the wait for someone you want to be with. I don't want to disrespect women. It's not that serious, and I won't let my hormones control me. I don't want to mess up someone else's future because of some short-term pleasure. My girlfriend and I both want to wait until marriage. Thanks for showing me the right way to go with life. I'm proud to say I can think with my head and not with my hormones.*
>
> **— High School Senior**

Check Your Hormones

I interviewed a 29-year-old once who had sex as a teenager. Yet, he and his wife dated for two and a half years and did not have sex until they married.

When I asked him how he abstained from sex during this time, he shared some things he did to keep his hormones in check:

- He and his wife never spent the night together while dating.
- He unfollowed women on social media whose posts he knew could cause him to have sexual thoughts.
- He skipped over sex scenes when watching movies.

And whenever he was where he felt his hormones were getting the best of him, he did the following:

- Worked out.
- Called accountability partners who knew he was abstaining so they could talk him off the ledge.

And if his accountability partners were not available, he would call someone else to serve as a distraction and take his mind off sex. Most times, he never even told them why he called. He just needed to focus on something other than his desire to have sex.

He is proof that your hormones do not have to control you.

The culture may have you believe otherwise. But, your hormones do not have the power to make you have sex unless you allow them to.

So ask yourself, who is in control? You or your hormones?

> *"You've motivated me to want to prove to myself that I control my hormones and my hormones don't control me."*
>
> **— High School Sophomore**

Reflection Questions

1 Do you think your hormones are at the same level when you are "kicking it" with your friends at the mall as they are if you are cuddled up on the couch making out? Why or why not?

2 How do you think the media you consume impacts your hormone levels?

3 Have you ever been where it was difficult to control your hormones? If so, what was going on at the time that caused your hormone levels to be high?

4 What are some limits/boundaries you can set to prevent yourself from getting to where your hormone levels get the best of you?

5 What are things you can do to avoid acting on your sexual urges if you get to where your hormones are getting the best of you?

#2

To relieve stress

When you said having sex may relieve stress temporarily, but it causes more stress afterwards, it hit me hard because that is so true for me.

— **High School Senior**

Some guys tell me they use sex to relieve stress, the same way they may play a game of basketball or get a massage. That may be true. But, sex only provides temporary relief. Yet, it can lead to much more stressful—and potentially permanent—consequences.

Whatever stress you may be attempting to relieve with sex, it is most likely nothing compared to an STD or a pregnancy. So why bother to reduce stress with an act that could cause even more later?

So why bother to reduce stress with an act that could cause even more later?

A high school senior shared his story with me after class one day. He discovered his girlfriend was pregnant during his junior year of high school. According to him, his father got upset if he brought a "B" home on his report card. So he could not imagine his father's reaction after discovering he would become a teen dad.

The thought of telling his dad was so stressful he could not do it. He told his older sister, who told his mom, who told his father.

The young man also said not having anyone to talk to about his stress caused him to fall into a deep depression. He searched for programs that help guys deal with teen pregnancy and could not find any. Which only added to his worries.

Find A Better Stress-Reliever

I am sure the stress this young man may have relieved during sex was not worth the stress he endured after his girlfriend became pregnant.

> *Your presentation made me realize a lot of things that could go wrong when you engage in sexual activity as a teen, from pregnancy to STD's. Your information helped me and my girlfriend in many ways. We used to worry about pregnancy almost every time. But since we have decided to*

> *stay away from sex, we have been happy and free from worries and stress. We have decided to wait till we are financially stable to support ourselves and maybe a baby. We'll also wait till marriage. We now know sex is not the key to happiness in a good relationship, but love and affection is the key. The key to safe sex is not to have sex till you have found the one that you will spend the rest of your life with.*
>
> **— High School Junior**

If you are stressed, it is clear that sex is not the answer. Instead, try to find activities that are productive rather than destructive. Pursue hobbies that will benefit your future rather than jeopardize it.

Practicing relaxation techniques with no strings attached is important. That way, you can destress without risking any harmful consequences down the road.

> *You came to our classroom a couple of days ago, and to be honest, before you even spoke, I was thinking about sex. But as you began discussing with us about the importance of abstinence, I realized that sex was more than just*

the stress-reliever people made it out to be. You made me realize that it was a commitment and also reminded me that with every commitment comes sacrifice and challenges. Now that you've shared your knowledge of abstinence to me, I am willing to face the sacrifices and challenges that come with abstinence.

— **High School Junior**

Self-Reflection Questions

1 Have any of your friends told you that sex was a great stress reliever? If so, what were your thoughts when they told you?

2 Why is stress relief a poor reason to have sex?

3 Do you know any guys who were stressed out after having sex due to an STD or pregnancy scare? What stressed them out? How did they handle the stress?

4 Have you ever thought about having sex to relieve stress? If so, what did you do? And what was the outcome?

5 What are 3 things you can do (other than sex) to relieve stress?

#3

Their friends have sex and they feel pressure to fit in

You said if your peers are sexually active, you may become active. Well, that's the only reason I'm not a virgin. I got pressured by my friends a lot. If I would have had peer support, I would still be a virgin.

— **High School Junior**

I get it. The pressure to have sex is REAL. Especially when it comes from your closest friends. Guys often tell me their friends pressure them to have sex, calling them lame, scared, etc., if they do not.

Negative Peer Pressure

Having sexually active friends contributes to guys' decisions to have sex. The desire to fit in often outweighs the best intentions to wait. And many guys will give in to the pressure, even knowing the potential consequences.

But here is the thing—like I tell the guys in my class, peer pressure does not have to be negative (which I will explain further a little later). And it will not be negative if friends are not having sex.

If you do not have friends who fit the bill, it might be time to make changes.

> *Recently, I've given in to a lot of peer pressure and had plans with friends to go out for what they consider a 'good time' as something they felt would serve to 'loosen me up.'*
> *I have now cancelled these plans. Sex is not what I should be looking for, you also reminded me of other goals in my life that are far more important.*
>
> **— High School Senior**

Internal Peer Pressure

There's pressure on me to have sex but it's not exactly from my friends. I apply pressure on myself to have sex because I see my friends doing it. And I'd like to be the one telling the story about my personal experience just once.

— High School Junior

Guys often pressure themselves to keep up with their peers. This peer pressure is not as obvious as friends shouting, "Do it! Do it! Do it!" It is much more subtle but can be every bit as damaging.

I am sure it's difficult to feel left out of discussions about sex or to feel like the only one not doing it. And yes, talking about girls and sex in the locker room may even help you "fit in."

But at what cost? Those friends will not be the ones dealing with potentially permanent consequences if . . .

1. your condom breaks,
2. her birth control fails,
3. or your partner has an STD she didn't mention.

> *At first, I thought abstaining
> from sex was lame.
> But you want to know what is
> really lame—having an STD.*
>
> — **High School Sophomore**

Positive Peer Pressure

This is why it is important to surround yourself with friends making good decisions. When most people hear about peer pressure, they typically assume it is negative. But, peer pressure can be positive if your influences are positive.

When I talked about positive vs. negative peer pressure in class one day, a senior guy said:

"That is so true about positive peer pressure. I am a virgin, and so are my three best friends. We hold each other accountable. I'm not sure I would still be a virgin if my three best friends were sexually active. And it would not necessarily be because they would have pressured me. If they were having sex, I would probably have put pressure on myself to start having sex so I could contribute to the conversation when they talked about what they were doing with their girlfriends."

If friends are making good decisions, then it is great to follow their example. Choosing friends who make positive choices eliminates unnecessary pressure you may have to deal with otherwise.

Self-Reflection Questions

1 Do you feel pressure to have sex? If so, does that pressure come from within or from your friends?

2 Which pressure is more difficult to handle? Internal pressure or peer pressure?

3 Why is it important to be selective about your choice of friends?

4 Do you have friends making good choices who challenge you to do the same? If so, who are they? If not, what friends should you pull back from so they do not impact your choices negatively?

5 What are three ways you can avoid internal and external peer pressure?

#4

To brag to their friends

At first, I thought having sex with a lot of girls was just for fun and something to brag about, but now I know there are life and death risks behind it.

— High School Junior

Having sex just to brag is a bad idea for several reasons. First, the people you brag to about sex—your friends—do not actually have anything of value to offer.

Those friends who care about your sex life cannot

1. get you into college,
2. give you a job,
3. or offer you anything for your long-term success.

Beyond that, they may not even be your friends ten years from now, so why make poor decisions to impress them? Why risk permanent consequences to get approval from temporary friends?

> *I lost my virginity when I was in the 8th grade. I had sex many more times. I only did it because I wanted to be cool, and yeah, I was cool for a minute, but I risked my life and hers, and that's more important than the sex.*
>
> **— High School Sophomore**

Your time might be better spent working to impress people who can help you with long-term success, like your parents, teachers, coaches or other adult role models. You impress them by hard work, discipline and passion—not by the number of girls you have slept with.

> *Many people, including myself, thought that it was cool to have sex with females and good for sharing stories with friends, basically bragging. Luckily, I haven't had sex and I don't plan on it until marriage, thanks to you.*
>
> **— High School Sophomore**

Why Teen Guys Brag

A friend and fellow speaker, Michael Calloway, shared the following with a group of teen girls one day:

> *Do you know why teen guys brag about having sex with girls? Because they know they got something they did not deserve. People do not brag about getting something they know they deserved or earned. How many people do you hear bragging when they get paid for working all week? I would venture to say few, if any, because they know they were not given anything they did not earn or deserve.*
>
> *There is a reason married men do not brag about having sex with their wives. A teen guy is the only person who brags to his friends about having sex because he knows he did not deserve what he got.*
>
> *Bragging is like a guy saying, "Can you believe this girl was willing to put her health, future, dreams and goals at risk for me—her silly boyfriend?"*

I am sure you are not the kind of guy who would allow a girl to put her health, future, dreams and goals at risk when you know you do not deserve her risking it all for you. Right?

I have found someone who loves me because even when I asked him how he felt about us not having sex yet, he said he would like to have sex; but he wanted to see me be the midwife I told him I wanted to be. And that he would be wrong if he held my hand and helped lead me down the wrong path.

— **High School Senior Girl**

Reflection Questions

1 Why do you think some guys brag about having sex or how many sexual partners they have had? Do you believe they are always telling the truth?

2 What are things you could be proud about accomplishing other than having sex?

3 Who are some people you would like to impress that could benefit you?

4 How long do you think the friendships you have now will last?

5 Do you think the friends you have now would pay for you to get treated for an STD or pay your child support? If so, who?

#5

They face pressure from their fathers and/or other adult men

To be honest, I never really considered abstinence. My whole life, my uncles and dad always teased me about having sex and all my cousins encouraged me to have sex.
Now that I've heard you speak, I realize I need to change.

— **High School Senior**

There is a prevailing attitude that teen boys should have sex, even when society expects teen girls to abstain. Men who expect their sons or boys in their community to have sex support this attitude. Which can translate into pressure on teen guys to become sexually active.

Because of this pressure, many young men will have sex to make their fathers and other adult men in their lives proud.

What Adult Men Don't Know Can Hurt You

It may seem these adult men are the ultimate authorities. But having sex because adults expect you to, does not make the consequences any less real. You may have more information about the risks of teenage sex than the adults in your life because the consequences are much more severe today than when they were teens.

When the men in your life were your age, their main concern might have only been preventing pregnancy and a few "treatable" STDs. Today, with 25+ STDs in existence, a pregnancy could be the least of your concerns.

Many adult men are not even aware there are incurable STDs spread by skin-to-skin contact that condoms cannot protect you from 100%.

Many men are also unaware that a test cannot be taken to determine whether they have the strain of human papillomavirus (HPV) that could give a woman cervical cancer.

So, ask yourself this: Do you want to risk taking the advice of someone pressuring you to have sex when they may not even realize the landmines you could face if you do?

I understand it may be difficult to deviate from the expectations of men you look up to. But, as Dr. Phil once said, "Sometimes you have to rise above your raising."

> *To me the most important thing that I learned was being able to rise above the way that I was raised. Because of the way that you repeated it, I was forced to think really hard about it and when I did, I understood why.*
>
> **— High School Sophomore**

When you know what is best for your health and your future, you have to overcome the expectations of those around you.

> *If there were more men in the world that taught the way that you do, then there wouldn't be so much pressure on the guys to feel like they're men just because they go out and put themselves at risk of hurting people that ultimately are the entire reason we are here. I want to be the father that can tell his son that you don't need sex to be popular, cool, or a man. Sincerely, A self-confident, reassured young MAN*
>
> **— High School Junior**

Self-Reflection Questions

1 Why do you think some men pressure boys to have sex?

2 Have you ever felt pressure from any of the adult men in your life to have sex? If so, what did they say or do to apply pressure?

3 If adult men have ever pressured you to have sex, do you know whether any of them experienced negative consequences because of having sex? If so, does that make you want to listen to their counsel?

4 Do you have a knowledgeable adult man you can go to for wise counsel about sex who will not pressure you to make choices that aren't in your best interests? If so, who?

5 Are there any cycles you need to break in your family related to sex and its consequences? If so, what are they and how will you break them?

#6

To satisfy curiosity

I agree sex before maturity is wrong, but I thought I would most likely lose my virginity just to fulfill my curiosity. I know, I sound really stupid, but unfortunately, most teens are thinking like this.

— **High School Freshman**

The young man who wrote this letter acknowledged that curiosity was a stupid reason to have sex, and he is not wrong.

This curiosity is usually motivated by the promise of pleasure that comes from sex. This is generally a bad idea, especially if you already know the associated risks. For example, curiosity about smoking, drugs and pornography can all lead to addiction.

Curiosity Isn't ALL Bad

Not that all curiosity is bad or that you should never explore new things. But no matter the scenario, taking considerable risks to explore a temporary pleasure is a poor choice. Having sex to find out about the pleasure, can lead you to discovering more than you ever wanted to know about the consequences.

So, if you are curious about sex, do yourself a favor and stay curious for a while. Teens often act like there is a ticking time bomb on their sex lives, but you have the rest of your life to find out about sex.

Why not save that curiosity until you are at a point where the risks of sex are lower? For example, when you are in a mutually monogamous, long-term, committed relationship where you know your partner's health history, trust them and would be okay if a pregnancy occurred.

Saving that curiosity can pay off in the end.

> *My girlfriend and I have been together for almost six months and like any young relationship, we started getting curious. After hearing you talk, I sat down with my girlfriend and explained how what we were doing could change our lives forever. The biggest influence on me was when you*

said, 'Would you want your daughter doing what you're doing with her boyfriend?' Personally, I would hurt someone that did that to my daughter, and it made me look at it because my girlfriend is someone's daughter. My girlfriend and I have put new boundaries in our relationship and we believe it will help, even if we don't stay together.

I wanna say thank you. If I hadn't heard your message, I might have been a father before I even got out of high school.

— High School Junior

Self-Reflection Questions

1 What do you think influences teens' curiosity about having sex?

2 Have you ever made a choice because you were curious, only to realize later it was a bad choice? If so, what was that choice and what were the consequences?

3 Why is curiosity NOT a good reason for teens to have sex?

4 On a scale of 1-10 (1 = not at all, 10 = very), how curious are you about having sex? And if you are no longer curious because you have had sex, was it worth the risk?

5 How could saving your curiosity about sex pay off for you in the end?

#7

To gain manhood

After listening to you, I talked to my boyfriend about what you said, and it made him rethink about having sex with me. My boyfriend is a virgin, and he wanted to have sex to prove he is a man, but in reality, he is not ready. We both decided to wait because neither of us wants to do it. I hope girls and boys understand that it's ok to be afraid, and that you shouldn't overwhelm yourself to do something you don't want to do.

— High School Junior Girl

Let's set the record straight right now—Manhood has NOTHING to do with having sex. I have heard stories of boys as young as 11 years old having sex. Clearly, an 11-year-old does not become a man because he does something anyone with functioning

Manhood has NOTHING to do with having sex.

Manhood is about having discipline and courage, making good decisions and taking care of responsibilities.

body parts can do. Sex does not make a boy a man. It makes him a boy blindly obeying his hormones.

Manhood is about having discipline and courage, making good decisions and taking care of responsibilities. NOT about having sex. With that settled, which one of these guys would get more of your respect as a man?

A 22-year-old college graduate, who just started a promising career, moved into his own apartment, looks forward to proposing to his girlfriend and is still a virgin?

OR

A 22-year-old who is unemployed after getting his ex-girlfriend pregnant, dropped out of high school and still lives with his parents, who help him support his 5-year-old son.

The True Measure of a Man

If sex was the criteria for manhood, the young man who became a teen father would be the obvious answer. Yet, the 22-year-old who is still a virgin has clearly demonstrated the traits necessary for manhood and should earn more respect.

So, if gaining manhood is your goal, sex is NOT the answer. Instead, focus on being disciplined, taking care of your responsibilities at home and at school, and making decisions that will honor your future wife and kids. That is what will make you a man.

> *The day after your presentation I was planning to have sex because I was being pressured. But when you spoke to our class, I saw that there are other guys out there that choose to be abstinent by choice. So, I saw that sex really wasn't the biggest thing out there. A real man doesn't need sex, a real man makes decisions that makes his life better and has the courage to say no.*
>
> **— High School Junior**

Self-Reflection Questions:

1 What do you think it means to be a man?

2 Why do you think so many people believe sex makes a boy a man?

3 Name 1–3 movies, songs, or television shows that send the message that sex makes you a man.

4 Would you rather be the virgin with the promising career about to propose to his girlfriend or the guy who was a teen father and may be having sex every day, but still living at home with his parents?

5 Have the choices you have made in the past with sex proven your manhood? Why or why not?

#8

The girls offer sex

You changed my life because I used to have sex with a new girl at least every three days. I never thought that only one time could cause so much harm. If you hadn't come, I would have probably gotten a disease or even gotten a girl pregnant. A lot of girls asked me to have sex with them and I said yes, like a fool. Now I will stay sex free until I am married.

— High School Senior

Some teen guys face external peer pressure to prove their manhood by having sex. And some young men have sex because it is offered and they think turning it down will make them look lame.

A lot of guys and girls will even say, "What kind of guy turns down sex?"

The correct answer?

A disciplined, thoughtful young man who values his health and his future. A young man who is strong enough to deny temporary pleasure for long-term benefits. But because of the expectations mentioned above, some guys may worry that refusing sex suggests there is something wrong with them.

When You Don't Want to Look Weak

A 15-year-old young man came to one of my mentees for advice. A young lady at his school offered to perform oral sex on him. Even though he did not want her to do it, he was not sure how to get out of it.

Since she had performed oral sex on many of his friends, he was afraid that he would look weak if he turned her down.

Denying sex does not make you weak. It makes you strong.

My mentee asked him to consider whether the risks he would be taking were worth not looking weak to people without his best interests at heart. Especially since he knew she had performed oral sex on many guys, which increased the chance, she could have an STD.

He also asked the young man if he had considered why any young lady would offer to perform oral sex on guys she was not even in a relationship with. Could it be that she may have some self-esteem issues?

My mentee challenged him to be a bigger man and not take advantage of her vulnerability.

If you remember nothing else from this book, remember this: Denying sex does not make you weak. It makes you strong.

And when it comes down to protecting your own future and health, who cares what anyone else thinks? Beyond that, a girl who does not recognize the value of a guy who is smart enough to abstain from sex, is a girl better off remaining in the "friend zone."

> *I have had sex before and every time I have had it, I have used a condom. Even though I wore a condom, I was still stressed out after doing it. My past two relationships were sex this, sex that. It wasn't me who really wanted to do it. It was my girlfriend. I regretted it, but I didn't want to make my girl mad. Ever since you came in, it has really taught me how to stick up for who I really am. I trust myself and I feel better about myself now.*
>
> **— High School Junior**

Self-Reflection Questions

1 Have you ever seen girls pressuring guys to have sex? If so, why do you think girls have become so aggressive with sex?

2 Would you have a problem telling a girl no if she tried to get you to have sex? What would be your fear of saying no?

3 How would you refuse a girl who asked you to have sex if you did not want to do it? What would you say to her?

4 Do you think saying yes to sex communicates that you and the young lady are in a relationship? Why or why not?

5 What are the dangers of having sex with someone who asks or pressures you to have sex when you are not even in a relationship?

#9

To experience physical pleasure

> *I'm 15 years old and I have been sexually active for a year now. I didn't care who I had sex with or how many girls. I just saw it as pleasure and having a good time. Like you said, it is pleasure for a moment; but after that, it's gone. I really am tired of sex. It's not worth it at all.*
>
> **— High School Sophomore**

This boy points out the primary problem with having sex for physical satisfaction—pleasure is fleeting. Yes, sex may feel good, but when it is over, you have to have sex again to get that same feeling.

Like drugs, the pleasure does not last and you get stuck in a cycle chasing the same short-term high. As we covered in the curiosity chapter, temporary pleasure is a bad reason to risk permanent consequences.

Over the summer, I had a chance to be with a girl I feel I'm in love with. Before it could happen though, I met with an old friend and we ended up having sex. Afterwards, I didn't feel like a man, but a lonely young boy afraid in the dark. I ended up telling the girl I'm in love with and she was devastated. She told me she never wanted to speak again. I was heartbroken. I still want to be with her, but I fear my past will haunt me forever because I sacrificed happiness for pleasure that felt like pain. I hope you share this letter, so everyone knows that sex is only pleasurable for the time that it lasts, and after, it's only a memory of pain and drama.

— **High School Junior**

Why should I risk ruining my—or someone else's—dreams and goals for something that is temporary, like pleasure. After all, we are teenagers. So why risk so much like our lives when most high school couples don't stay together?

— **High School Sophomore**

A young lady said one day, "I told my boyfriend what you said about sex and he said that you did not know what you were talking about. So he asked why you did not talk about any of the good parts of sex."

I said, "I am sure he thinks sex feels good. Well, crack feels good to a crack addict. The question is, 'Is it doing you any good?'"

Facts vs. Feelings

You can make your decisions based on one of two things—facts or feelings. Feelings change. Facts don't! The feeling you get from sex is very temporary.

The fact is it is never the best choice for teens to have sex. That was a fact yesterday. That is a fact today. And it will be a fact tomorrow.

You can make your decisions based on one of two things— facts or feelings. Feelings change. Facts don't!

Yet, the prevailing attitude in our society is, "If it feels good, do it." If you subscribe to that philosophy, you may end up unfulfilled as an adult and saying to yourself, "There has to be more to life than this." And you would be right.

There are things in life that give permanent satisfaction and genuine fulfillment. Things like doing work you love or mentoring a child from an underprivileged household.

In either case, there is not a paycheck or a "thank you" that could ever measure up to the sense of fulfillment you receive. Instead, you are a part of something bigger than yourself.

Sex and other temporary pleasures are fake versions of real satisfaction and fulfillment. They are like giving someone a candy bar once a week as opposed to full meals every day.

There is so much more to life than sex. I challenge you right now as a teen to spend time discovering what "more" there is for your life.

Go beyond what feels good *to* you to what is good *for* you!

You changed the way I think about sex. I used to think sex was just something that gave me pleasure, but now I don't want short-term pleasure to ruin my life or my future child's life. You've opened my eyes about what sex really is. It's not just pleasure, but a commitment. A commitment to a possible STD. A commitment to a baby that might come whether you like it or not. Before this, my mind was screaming sex, sex, sex, but now it's saying slow down, wait, you can handle it. I just want to thank you for giving a clearer definition on sex. I have basketball and school to focus on. Sex will come later.

— High School Senior

Self-Reflection Questions:

1 How do you think the temporary pleasure you would get from having sex would compare to the long-term consequences that could result from it?

2 What are things that could come with the pleasure of sex?

3 Why do you think our culture promotes the "YOLO—You Only Live Once" mentality regarding decision-making?

4 Have you ever chosen to do something you knew would only bring you temporary pleasure even though there were risks involved? If so, what was it?

5 What type of pleasure can come from abstaining from sex?

#10

They are embarrassed about being a virgin

I had sex once before I saw you. The honest reason was a bad one. I just wanted the title of virgin off of me.
So, I saw the chance and took it. Before you came, all I thought about was sex, which probably isn't a surprise considering I'm a 16-year-old boy.
But after hearing you speak, my mindset changed.

— High School Junior

A 10th grader approached me after an assembly one day. Even though he was a virgin he lied and told his friends he was not. He said if his friends knew he was still a virgin, they would make fun of him.

I told him that abstaining was one of the best decisions he could make to protect his future. And he should allow no one to make him feel ashamed for making a good choice.

And if he ever admitted to his friends he was a virgin, I gave him advice on what to say if they teased him... "I can do what you are doing any day of the week; but can you do what I am doing?"

"Virgin" is NOT A Bad Word

I heard a male friend share the following story with an audience of all teen guys . . .

He said when he was in high school, all his friends bragged about having sex. He was a virgin and hated that he could never contribute to the conversation.

To get the title of "virgin" off of him, he had sex with someone he was not even dating. And could not wait to go back and share with the guys about having had sex.

Years later, after they all left for college, the subject came up in conversation. His friends were shocked to discover he actually had sex in high school. They assumed he was lying about it like they were.

Imagine that. They were ALL lying about having sex.

And since none knew that the others were lying, my friend had sex so he would not be the only virgin, only to find out that they had not had sex either.

Thankfully, he suffered no physical consequences because of a decision he only made to fit in with guys who were lying about their sexual choices too.

How tragic it would have been if he had gotten the girl pregnant or contracted an STD. And somehow, I doubt his buddies would have been around to help out if he had.

So, if you ever hang out with your boys talking about who is sexually active, consider this . . .

Why allow someone too weak to control his own hormones make you feel bad because you are strong enough to control yours? It takes a much stronger person to say no to sex than it does to say yes, and that choice pays off in the long run.

It frees you up to focus on your goals. You also do not have to worry about unplanned pregnancies, STD's or the drama that often accompanies teenage sexual relationships.

> *You made me realize the choices that I was about to make were the wrong ones. I was the guy that was still a virgin, but bragged about doing it. I told my friends I wasn't so I wouldn't feel left out from the group and conversations they had. This urged me to want to lose my virginity sooner. After your presentation, you have given me more confidence in myself and showed me that holding myself to a higher standard is*

much more important than worrying about what people think about me being a virgin.

— **High School Junior**

Self-Reflection Questions:

1 Have you ever felt embarrassed for people to know you were a virgin? If so, why?

2 Have you ever lied about having sex? Why or why not?

3 Who do you think guys would be most embarrassed by them discovering they are a virgin? Friends, fathers, girls, etc.? Why or why not for each?

4 Do you know any teen guys who admit to being a virgin? If so, did you tease them about it or think less of them?

5 How does being a virgin show strength vs. being sexually active?

Conclusion

Wait or have sex? The choice is yours! Not mine. Not your peers'. Not even your parents can decide for you.

After reading this book, I hope you will not only have decided to wait, but will understand your reasons.

Knowing your "why" is what will help you wait when your friends are bragging about having sex and you are once again left out of the conversation.

When your hormones seem to plot against you and your resolve to wait.

Or when the girl of your dreams says she wants to take your relationship to the next level.

Without a "why" you will not wait. So, take the time to figure out what yours is.

To make it easier, you now have 10 great reasons to abstain from sex:

1. You know your value
2. To be a protector and not a predator
3. You have discipline and self-control
4. You love and respect women
5. To be a role model for your younger siblings, especially your sister(s)

6. To protect your future child(ren)
7. To protect your future spouse
8. To avoid negative consequences
9. You have dreams and goals
10. You are proud of who you are and your decisions

Choose one, three or all ten, and enjoy the relief and pride that comes with waiting.

You will be glad you did!